HAIR LOSS CURE

A Revolutionary Hair Loss Treatment You Can Use At
Home To Grow Your Hair Back!

By
GAL RUBIN

TABLE OF CONTENTS

INTRODUCTION

In this step-by-step process you will systematically remove all of the factors that are causing your hair to stop growing. While you are eliminating the causes of your hair loss you will be increasing the influence of factors that encourage your hair to grow and prevent hair loss.

In this short e-book, I will provide detailed instructions on how to perform at-home procedures that eliminate each of the root causes of hair loss. It also explains why you are doing the things you are doing. These procedures have been refined over many years, to produce the ultimate hair growth methodology.

In order to explain the reasoning behind certain instructions I have had to use some specialist terminology, such as 'DHT', 'sebum', 'alopecia', and 'alopecia areata'. Some of you will recognize this terminology, while others will not but we will go into further detail in the pages to come.

In steps 1+2, I will explain exactly what to do to prepare the scalp so that new hairs can actually start growing again, and existing hairs will become stronger.

Without the scalp preparation it's much harder for new hairs to grow because where the hair follicle exits, the skin has become blocked, clogged, and the pH is generally very unfavorable for new hair growth.

In step 3, I will explain how to reactivate the hair growth process using a little known technique that initiates the growth phase of the hair follicle. And finally I will show you how to stimulate the scalp and emerging hair follicles in such a way that they continue to grow, faster and stronger.

Please take your time with the instructions. Don't rush. Incorporating change into your life should be done thoughtfully and carefully. Our how to prevent hair loss guide has a lot to take in but just take it one step at a time. Don't try to do it all at once. Each step will make a positive difference for your hair loss treatment.

Please try your best follow the instructions as closely as possible every day for six months. If you can maintain that commitment you will not regret it. I believe this is one of the most effective method in the world for preventing hair loss (with the exception of a hair transplant). This method eliminates every underlying cause of hair loss without the use of drugs to alter hormonal balance.

WARNINGS

Do not under any circumstances follow the instructions in this website that advise you to make changes to your diet if you are pregnant or breastfeeding. If you are on medication or have a medical condition you must consult your doctor before applying any of the instructions contained in this book for your own safety. If you have any concerns about applying any of the instructions please email us at: hairloss.office@gmail.com.

It is strongly recommended that you consult your doctor before beginning any supplementation program as he or she will have an understanding of your medical history. If you experience any side-effects as a result of using supplements please cease usage immediately and consult your doctor. If you are pregnant, lactating or using any medications, please consult your doctor before using supplements.

DISCLAIMER

All content within this e-book is provided for general information only, and should not be treated as a substitute for the medical advice of your own doctor or any other health care professional. Howtopreventhairloss.ca is not responsible or liable for any diagnosis made by a user based on the content of this website. The author is not liable for the contents of any external internet sites listed, nor does it endorse any commercial product or service mentioned or advised on the website. Always consult your own GP if you're in any way concerned about your health.

STEP 1: EXFOLIATING THE SCALP

In this step, I will show you how to increase hair growth by exfoliating your scalp with a hard bristle boar brush. Your hair receives the nutrients it needs to grow through the bloodstream .

If you show signs of baldness, thinning hair, or alopecia - then a simple scalp exfoliation can help by increasing the blood supply to your hair follicles.

Your hair receives the nutrients it needs to grow via the bloodstream. If your hair is weak, brittle, lackluster or thinning, it is almost certainly not receiving a good blood supply .

However, we can fix this (ie. scalp exfoliation), and many of the instructions in this guide on how to prevent hair loss. The better the blood supply to your hair follicles, the more hair growth you will see. We need to do everything we can to increase the blood supply to your hair follicles.

Years of using conditioners, gels, waxes, hair sprays and other cosmetics may have caused a build-up of chemicals on your scalp. We need to exfoliate your scalp to make the skin fresh, healthy and the pores clear. Let's start with a simple mild exfoliation:

HARD BRISTLED BOAR BRUSH

Purchase a hard bristled boar brush which will cost you between $1 and $20.

I strongly recommend buying a good quality one (with real, tough boar hairs) as it will last ten times as long and will exfoliate your scalp more effectively.

THE EXERCISE:

You should perform it between three and five times per day for about 2 minutes, every day. If you you have fragile hair that is susceptible to split ends, consider applying a small amount of pure coconut oil to your hair half an hour before doing the exfoliation, to protect your hair. Only use a very small amount of coconut oil and apply it to your hair, not your scalp.

As you progress through this website, your hair will get much stronger. Even the boar brush technique will increase the strength of your hair.

Once every few weeks, give your brush a good wash. If you're using the coconut oil to protect your hair, wash the brush every day. From time to time wash the brush with a little antibacterial spray and rinse very well.

Please note: If you have a flaky or inflamed scalp, don't complete Step 1 yet. Instead, Consult a medical professional first.

HOW TO PERFORM THE EXERCISE:

Make sure your hair is dry. Don't perform this exercise if your hair is wet.

Brush your scalp 100 times, holding the brush firmly down to scrape the scalp skin, exfoliating it .

Brush your scalp in one direction – either back to front, or front to back. This should not be painful.

If you notice your scalp feeling a little sensitive, stop doing the boar brush exfoliation for the remainder of the day .

No Be aware: You may notice a little sensitivity due to Dermaroller use (you'll learn about the Derma roller in later steps). If so, go a bit easier on the brushing. While you are doing this you can start your hair growth nutrition program.

STEP 2: SCALP PEEL FOR HAIR RE-GROWTH

In this step, we are going to talk about a new hair growing tip by doing a simple scalp skin peel .

Using this simple peel, we will essentially aim to strip away years of built up cosmetics, pollutants, dead skin cells and sebum from your scalp, clearing the pores and completely renewing your scalp. This scalp skin peel will get your scalp back into the condition it was before you had signs of baldness or alopecia .

By the end of this step your scalp should be fresh and ready to make hair grow faster than ever before.

Preparing the scalp means cleaning it, removing both the natural and unnatural substances that have built up there, which are both the cause and effect of hair loss.

Without the cleaning process, new hairs are less likely to appear because they literally have to push and squeeze their way out of the epidermis, and this makes it less likely to happen. It's like a plant that has to grow through a thick layer of gravel that's dry and acidic, even if there is fertile ground beneath, it has a much harder task.

Our aim is to make it as easy as possible for new hair growth to occur.

So what should be cleaned from the epidermis to allow hair growth? Well there are 4 things we have to remove first. These are;

1. Embedded sebum

2. Dead skin

3. Cosmetic products

4. Pollutants

These 4 substances will become mixed together and form what's called epidermis plaque that clings to the scalp and prevents hair growth and causes miniaturization of existing hair follicles.

The plaque also contains DHT that's secreted through the epidermis creating a perpetually inhospitable environment for hair growth.

By doing the salicylic acid peel, we are going to strip away years of built up cosmetics, pollutants, dead skin cells and embedded sebum from your scalp, clearing the pores and completely renewing your scalp .

The objective of this process is to get your scalp back into the condition it was in before you started losing your hair. By the end of this step your scalp should be fresh and the pores should be unclogged, providing the perfect environment for hair growth.

WHAT IS 'SEBUM' AND WHY SHOULD YOU CLEAN IT?'

Sebum is the oil that secretes through your skins pores via the sebaceous gland. Dead skin cells, sebum, cosmetics and air pollutants can combine and build-up on the scalp and in the pores.

Ideally we want to take off several layers of skin during this step; but don't worry, the scalp is very thick and we're only going to exfoliate a tiny fraction of the skin – taking away dead skin cells, pollutants, built-up cosmetic chemicals and built-up sebum.

"Apart from the balls of the feet, the heels and back, it's (the scalp is) the thickest part of the skin. The top layer, or epidermis is of average thickness but the dermis, which is the stronger layer of

skin underneath, is thicker. Whereas facial skin may measure 1mm, the skin on the scalp is about 2mm ".

•DR CHRISTOPHER ROWLAND PAYNE, CONSULTANT DERMATOLOGIST AT THE LONDON CLINIC

To begin with we're going to do something that may seem quite extreme, but is a very powerful technique for improving the long term health of your scalp and hair .

What we're going to do next is apply a mild, natural acid to your scalp, in order to break up the dead skin from the surface of the scalp, clear your scalp's pores, kill mites and fungi that may be present in your scalp and break down embedded sebum.

HOW TO REMOVE THE EMBEDDED SEBUM BASED PLAQUE

The best way to remove embedded sebum from your scalp and to clear the pores is to use a 'salicylic acid peel' product .

These peels are commonly used to reduce the appearance of wrinkles, clear the skins pores and reveal younger looking skin .

Salicylic acid was originally used to exfoliate the skin to make it younger. We're going to use the same skin peels that are used on the face to exfoliate your scalp .

It's safe to use this mild acid on the scalp because the hair follicle roots grows from much deeper in the scalp then the acid reaches so it won't cause hair loss in any way.

However, you should not complete a scalp peel if you have a flaky or inflamed scalp.

SAFETY WARNING

While it is perfectly safe to use salicylic acid on your skin, please do not stray from these safety warnings:

Do not leave the salicylic acid on your scalp for more than twenty minutes

Always leave at least ten days between completing skin peels

If you feel a strong stinging sensation on your scalp after applying the salicylic acid, wash it out immediately

If your skin becomes irritated or peels a lot (you see lots of skin flakes a day or two after completing the peel) do not complete another peel

Do not complete more than three peels within a month. If you complete three peels within a month, leave at least two months before completing another.

After completing a skin peel, you should not notice any significant peeling of your skin. You should not see lots of flaky skin and your skin should not feel painful. In fact nine times out of ten you won't notice any change in your skin after completing the peel, except perhaps a little flakiness a day or two after completing the peel.

THE SALICYLIC ACID PEEL:

First of all you need to purchase some salicylic acid; you can buy salicylic acid skin peel products online. To begin with, choose a product with a 10% concentration of salicylic acid. You can purchase a bottle online on eBay or from many health and beauty stores.

SALICYLIC ACID FOR HAIR

Salicylic acid can be used to clean the scalp and remove DHT. Before you use salicylic acid it's recommended to do a skin test to make sure you're not allergic to it. This involves applying a small amount of the solution to a visible piece of skin.

You will also benefit from using a very small amount of the coconut oil you purchased for eating when you drink your smoothies. We're going to use coconut oil to protect the hair from damage during the peel. Although the acid will not damage your hair, the alcohol in the peel solution may have a slight drying effect on your hair. The coconut oil prevents any 'protein loss' from the hair.

The ability of coconut oil to penetrate into hair cuticle and cortex seems to be responsible for this effect. Coated on the fibre surface, it can prevent or reduce the amount of water penetrating into the fibre and reduce the swelling. This, in turn, reduces the lifting of the surface cuticle and prevents it from being chipped away during wet combing.

•Aarti S. Rele and R. B. Mohile, The Journal of Cosmetic Science, April 2002

Before applying the acid to your scalp, apply coconut oil to your hair to form a protective coating. You'll learn how to do this when we get on to the peel process. First though you need to do a 'skin test.'

BEGINNING THE FIRST FULL SCALP PEEL

Once you're happy with the test peel results you can start your first full scalp peel. At least half an hour before beginning the peel, apply the coconut oil to your hair, as follows:

Thoroughly wash your hair and scalp and dry with a towel to remove any dampness (it doesn't need to be bone dry but make sure it's not damp). Apply a very small amount of coconut oil to your hair to coat the base 2-3 inches of hair. Run your fingers through your hair and rub the coconut oil in .

Don't massage the coconut oil into your scalp – avoid getting the coconut oil on your scalp as much as possible, as this will act as a barrier between the acid and the skin. Ideally you should wait roughly 30 minutes or more for the coconut oil to absorb into your hair.

Once you're happy that you've coated your hair with coconut oil and you've left enough time for it to absorb, you can start to apply the acid to your scalp. The best way to apply the salicylic acid to your scalp is with a pipette. You may find that your product comes with a pipette. If not you can purchase them online on eBay for less than a dollar per pack.

LET'S BEGIN THE PEEL

If you have short hair, spike your hair up. If you have long hair, part your hair down the middle. If you have shaven hair, very thin hair or no hair you will have no trouble applying the acid. If you need to part your hair to access your scalp with the pipette you will need to apply the acid to the parted area, then part your hair again to the left and right of the middle parting two or three times until you have covered your scalp in little droplets of salicylic acid.

Fill the pipette with acid from the bottle. Point the pipette downward without pinching it – make sure none of the acid drips out. Now, touch the end of the pipette onto your scalp and gently squeeze so that a very small drop comes out onto your scalp. Elevate the pipette, move it half an inch or so away from the first drop and squeeze another small drop onto your scalp. Repeat this process until you have about 40-50 small drops of acid spread out across the top of your scalp, without pouring any onto your hair. You should be able to do this in a few minutes – you can squeeze out two or three droplets per second, so the process should only take a few minutes. You will inevitably get some acid on your hair but don't worry; it won't damage your hair. Salicylic acid is used to break down oils and skin tissue but at this concentration it will not damage your hair.

Once you've covered your scalp with small droplets, rub the acid in with your fingers until it covers the top of your scalp and then wash your hands. The acid will not damage your hands at this concentration, but wash them as soon as you've finished rubbing the acid into your scalp. Leave the peel on for one minute. You should feel a very mild stinging sensation, or a cool tingling sensation. This is normal and means the peel is working. However if you feel a painful stinging sensation, wash the acid out immediately.

If after one minute the acid feels like it's burning (stinging quite badly), wash it out. If it's still not stinging after one minute then leave it in for ten minutes. If it's still not stinging after ten minutes, wash it out. If it starts to sting uncomfortably before ten minutes, wash it out. Many people find that the acid stings their scalp for around thirty seconds and then the stinging dies down. If you find this occurs, leave the acid on for ten minutes and then wash it out.

To wash the acid out, first rinse your hair and scalp with water for about a minute while gently rubbing your scalp with your fingers. Then wash your scalp by massaging with shampoo and rinsing. Directly after completing the peel, drink a pint of water. Some salicylic acid may absorb into your skin. This is nothing to worry about and is common during normal face skin peels. However it is good practice to drink lots of water during the day you complete the peel.

INCREASE EXFOLIATION AFTER COMPLETING THE PEEL
You can help increase the exfoliation by brushing your scalp with your hard bristled boar brush, as described in Step 1. To do this brush your scalp firmly about fifty times (or for about a minute)

each day starting from two days after completing the peel. For the two days immediately following completing the peel don't use the boar brush and don't apply any chemicals to your scalp (such as minoxidil for example). Give your scalp a chance to reject and remove the dead skin cells. After two days you can continue to use the boar brush and any other treatments you might be using, such as minoxidil.

ACHIEVING A SUCCESSFUL PEEL

If the peel has worked you should notice your scalp turn flaky a day or two after completing the peel. You can help exfoliate the dead skin flakes by brushing them away using the brush .

This process can seem counter-intuitive to someone who suffers hair loss because you're stripping away skin from your scalp and it seems like you're doing damage rather than good. Actually it's hugely beneficial because you're unclogging pores, removing dirt and pollutants and getting your scalp skin into a fresh clean state, ready for hair growth.

NEW PLAQUE BUILD-UP

It varies from person to person but there's a good chance you will need another few peels to fully remove the plaque. Repeat the procedure until you feel like the plaque has been removed. You can aid the process by brushing away the flakes that fall off with a hairbrush, which also helps de-clog the pores.

You might find that the plaque builds up quickly again; this is because of the overproduction of the sebum that debilitates hair growth

Ok that's the procedure for preparing the scalp for new hair growth. Let's summarize it quickly

Test the salicylic acid on your skin

Monitor the results to make sure no adverse reactions occur

Wash and dry hair, apply coconut oil to hair strands

Apply salicylic acid to scalp using pipette

Rinse with warm water after ten minutes, or 30 seconds after mild stinging sensation.

Rinse immediately if painful

SUMMARY TO STEP 2:

To summarize what we've done in Step 2. We have:

- Peeled the top layers of scalp skin

- Unblocked any blocked pores on the scalp

- Removed some of the DHT from the scalp

- Removed built-up embedded sebum

- Helped kill mites if they were present

Provoked the body to concentrate healing in the scalp by: increasing blood circulation in the scalp (increasing blood supply to the hair roots), increasing cell production in the scalp, increasing nutrient supply to the scalp

Now we need to move on to a more advanced treatment, where we'll feed the hair with an abundance of nutrients required for hair growth and continue to provoke your body to concentrate cell growth, blood circulation and nutrient allocation in the scalp.

STEP 3: REACTIVATING HAIR FOLLICLES

In this step I will show you how to help your alopecia and increase hair growth by reactivating dormant hair follicles. This is another great home remedy for hair growth and helping with your baldness or alopecia .

We are going to use the alternation method which will mildly and temporarily damage the scalp and then encourage rapid healing through use of a special hair growth tonic.

We initially need to activate the hair follicles and epidermis from their dormant state, wake them up and send a signal to your body that says 'hey it's beneficial to use our resources to grow hair right now.'

We need to put them into a state of activity by telling the body to send all the building blocks for hair growth tasks.

Without activating the scalp, much of our hard work will go into repairing and building other parts of the body that are in need. (This definitely isn't a bad thing at all, but for our purposes we can 'trick' our bodies to send its supplies into the scalp for new hair growth).

For this we'll need a derma-roller. This is a device like a rolling pin, except that this one is covered in hundreds of tiny needles about 0.5mm long. The dermaroller is rolled across the scalp it produces thousands of tiny pricks in the epidermis.

The pricks aren't deep enough to do any long-term damage; they're just deep enough to wake up the cells in that area so they can send their resources. This helps increase cell production and circulation to the epidermis.

THE ALTERNATION METHOD

The alternation method uses a special technique that mildly (and temporarily) damages the scalp and then encourages rapid healing through use of a special hair growth tonic. By mildly damaging the scalp we encourage increased blood circulation right at the surface of the scalp, increasing the supply of nutrients to the hair which in turn will reactivate hair follicles and increase hair growth.

We then use a special topical hair growth tonic to directly feed the hair and protect the scalp. The result is that dormant hair follicles receive a massive increase of nutrients, triggering them to start re-growing.

We need a special tool for this called a 'Dermaroller.'

THE DERMAROLLER

A Dermaroller is a small rolling pin type device, which is covered in tiny metal needles.

It is designed to heal scars and is often used to reduce the appearance of stretch marks, scars resulting from surgery and acne scars .

This device was originally meant to be used to promote younger skin and heal acne wounds, stretch marks and scars. The roller pricks stimulate the new growth of collagen and elastin fibres, as well as new melanozytes, and re-vascularization.

The tiny wounds heal in less than an hour, but the cells remain stimulated. In a way it's similar to pruning a bush, or cutting the grass. Where the cut was made, growth hormones flood to, and fresh vegetation growth can be found soon after. It's important to clean the roller each time you use it to prevent any chance of infection.

You can do this by washing in boiling hot water, or a mild antibacterial solution before use.

For hair growth purposes, we are going to use the principles of the Dermaroller to encourage increased cell production and increased circulation in the scalp .

When you combine this with the use of some special ingredients that feed your hair, you will increase hair growth and reactivate dormant hair follicles – thus increasing the density of your hair .

You can purchase A dermaroller on eBay for around $20 (The needle size you need is a minimum of 0.5mm to a max of 1 mm). If you want a bundle of a derma roller, dermastamp and the hair tonic – feel free to email us and place an order.

USING THE DERMAROLLER TO ACTIVATE HAIR GROWTH

Lightly roll the dermaroller over the parts of your scalp suffering from hair loss. Apply just enough pressure that the tiny needles penetrate the skin. You might feel a tingling sensation but it shouldn't hurt.

Go over the effected parts of your scalp 4 times each at a different angle each time, covering all of the top of your scalp .

Go over the every part of your scalp four times (as shown in the diagram above), making sure to cover all of your scalp – you don't need to go over the back and sides of your head, just the top, where the hair loss is occurring. Concentrate more on the areas of your hair that are thinning most.

After you've done this, you can now apply the special hair growth tonic.

FREQUENCY OF USING A DERMA ROLLER

You should apply the derma-roller and tonic every other day to start with. Once your scalp has got use to it, you can do it every day, or however often you feel it will be beneficial and convenient to you. Once a day after a few weeks seems to work well.

Do it before bed, this gives the maximum time to heal without interruption.

THE CUSTOM HAIR GROWTH TONIC:

As well as using the Dermaroller several times a week, you are going to make your own custom Hair Growth Tonic, to help directly feed your hair, protect your hair and scalp and to reverse damage caused by DHT.

I'm not talking about minoxidil either, this is much cheaper and much more effective. This formula came about through a series of trial and error with myself and a lot of research, so please make the most of it

THE INGREDIENTS OF THE HAIR GROWTH TONIC:

Emu oil

Borage (starseed) oil

Apple polyphenols supplement

High strength saw palmetto soft gels

Magnesium oil (from a sea source(

Tea Tree oil

The easiest way to find the products needed for the Hair Growth Tonic is to search through eBay.

HOW TO MIX THE HAIR GROWTH FORMULA:

Purchase a small bottle (such as a 60 ml bottle)

Add about 18 ml of Emu Oil.

Add about 18 ml of Borage Oil.

Add about 20 drops of Tea Tree Oil and shake well.

Now break open 10 polyphenols capsules and pour the powder into the bottle. Shake well.

Next pierce 10-15 saw palmetto soft gels with a sharp knife tip and pour/squeeze the oil into the bottle. Shake well.

Optionally add several pinches of cayenne pepper.

Finally, fill the remainder of the bottle with the magnesium oil.

Lastly, Shake well.

**Based on a 60ml bottle size follow these instructions.

Now you have what is probably one of the most effective hair growth topicals on the planet.

HOW TO APPLY THE HAIR GROWTH TONIC

Before using the Hair Growth Tonic all over your scalp, it is advisable to do a test patch overnight to see how your skin reacts. If you've used hair gel, hair wax or other styling products in your hair during the day, wash your hair and scalp before using the Dermaroller. Make sure your hair is clean and dry before using the Dermaroller.

NOW APPLY THE HAIR GROWTH TONIC

After using the Dermaroller, squeeze several blobs of the Hair Growth Tonic onto your scalp and massage it into the skin really well. Slowly massage the tonic deeply into your scalp. The tonic will absorb into your scalp, feeding and nourishing your hair follicles.

Over the next 24 hours your scalp may be just the slightest bit uncomfortable – although this will hardly be noticeable .

That's ok, each time you repeat the process the uncomfortable feeling will get less. If you feel strong discomfort, wash the mixture away with warm water.

The needle punctures heal very quickly and this process does wonders for your hair.

Wait 24 hours and look out for any signs of reaction. (This has never happened to anyone I know, but just in case(

Be sure to wash out the hair growth tonic with a high quality ORGANIC shampoo.

 **Very Important:

You must clean your Derma Roller after every use Using alcohol.

FINAL WORDS

You have to persevere with this method to get the most out of it. If you do it half-heartedly and irregularly then the results will probably not be satisfactory.

However, if you carry it out as instructed, along with the other steps, in my experience, there is no hair treatment (aside from a direct hair transplant) that gets as good results.

If you are using Minoxidil then substitute this mixture for it. The side effects of minoxidil will go away, and only natural ingredients will reach the scalp. It's also much less expensive.

GOOD LUCK!